How I Became A

VETERINARIAN

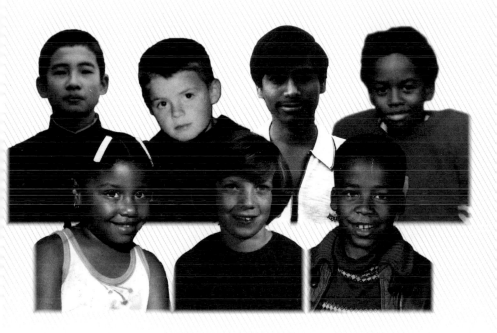

"How I Became A Veterinarian"

Written by:
Sandy Amass, DVM, PhD, DABVP
Kauline Davis, PhD
Paula Green, M.Ed., NCC, NCSC

Designed by:
Thad Blossom, BS

Reviewed by:
Adrianne Fisch, BS
Ann Mennonno, MS
Dorothy Reed, PhD
Amy Wackerly, BS (Sports Mgmt.), BS (Elem. Ed.)

Summary:
Meet veterinarians from all over the
world who make sure animals stay healthy.

Special thanks to our Purdue Veterinarians:
Laurent Couëtil, DVM, PhD, DACVIM
Henry Green, III, DVM, DACVIM
Tomo Inoue, DVM
Yava Jones, DVM, PhD, DACVP
Willie Reed, DVM, PhD, DACVP, DACPV
Ramesh Vemulapalli, BVSc, MVSc, PhD
Tracy Vemulapalli, DVM, MS, DACLAM

This book is part of the "Fat Dogs and Coughing Horses: Animal Contributions towards a Healthier Citizenry" program at Purdue University. Fat Dogs and Coughing Horses is made possible by Science Education Partnership Award (SEPA) funding from the National Institutes of Health (NIH).

Table of Contents

<u>Chapter One</u>

The Walrus and the Pinecone

by Sandy Amass

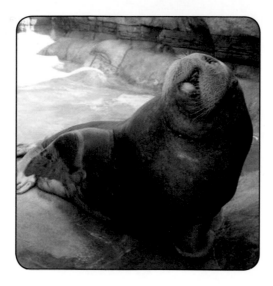

Caesar is a walrus who lives at the zoo. He weighs 2,800 pounds! He is usually a happy walrus who loves to eat. Walruses use their whiskers to dig and find clams and other food from the bottom of the sea floor. They are curious about new things and will eat anything they find. This is a problem because their stomachs can only digest fish or squid. They cannot digest plants. One day, Caesar did not feel well. He did not want to swim. He did not want to eat. Caesar had an upset stomach.

The veterinary team was called to help Caesar. They examined Caesar and decided that he must have eaten something that he shouldn't have. The veterinary team decided to do surgery to find out what was in Caesar's stomach that was making him sick. They decided to do surgery the next day.

Dr. Tomo Inoue is a veterinarian. He is an anesthesiologist. He makes sure that animals, like Caesar, stay asleep during surgery and don't feel any pain. Today was going to be a big day. Dr. Tomo was part of the veterinary team helping Caesar. Dr. Tomo is also a husband and a father. His wife, Dr. Stephanie, is a veterinarian. They have twins, a boy and a girl. On the morning of Caesar's surgery, Dr. Tomo woke up at 6:00 a.m. and got his kids ready for day care. They dressed, ate breakfast and left home by 6:30 a.m. Dr. Tomo took his kids to day care and then drove to the zoo.

Dr. Tomo arrived at the zoo to get Caesar ready for surgery. Caesar needed a shot to make him sleepy, but Caesar was grouchy and did not want anyone to touch him. Dr. Tomo blew through a long tube to shoot a dart into Caesar's muscle. The dart contained medicine to make Caesar sleepy. Once Caesar was sleepy, Dr. Tomo put a face mask on him. The mask was hooked to a machine that delivered anesthesia to keep Caesar asleep during surgery.

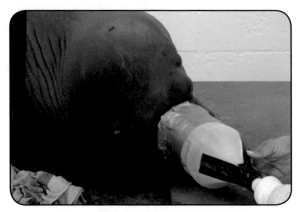

Animals that live in the water, like walruses, can hold their breath for a very long time. For the anesthesia to work, it was important that Caesar did not hold his breath. Part of Dr. Tomo's job was to make sure that Caesar kept breathing during the surgery. Once Caesar was sound asleep, a veterinary surgeon opened up his stomach and found what was making Caesar sick. He had eaten a pinecone! The surgeon removed the pinecone and when Caesar woke up, he felt great!

Where did the pinecone come from? There was a pine tree near Caesar's pool. The pinecone must have fallen into the water. The zookeepers quickly put a net over Caesar's pool so no more pinecones could fall in and make Caesar sick. They also put a sign up asking visitors to not feed the animals. Now, no more walruses would get sick from eating something they should not eat. Dr. Tomo was happy. It was a great day! He went home to see his wife and kids, ate dinner, and went to sleep smiling.

Meet Dr. Tomo Inoue

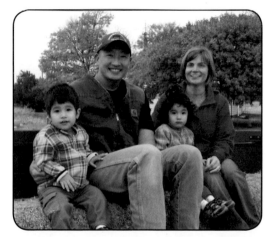

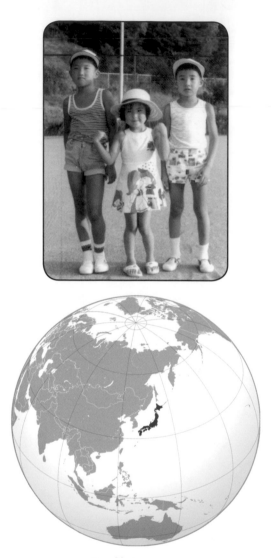

Growing up

Dr. Tomo grew up in Osaka, Japan. He lived in Japan until he was 20 years old. Osaka is the second largest city in Japan. Dr. Tomo has an older brother and a younger sister. He is the middle child. His parents live in Osaka. His dad is a physician (a doctor for people). His mom is a nurse.

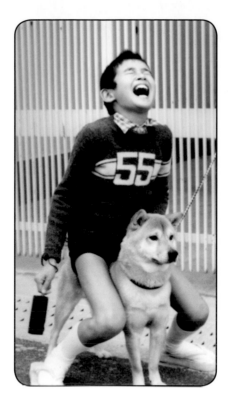

Pets

Dr. Tomo grew up around animals. His family had two cats, two dogs, fish, salamanders, birds, turtles, lizards and giant beetles. His favorite thing to do on summer vacation was to go into the woods in the evening and put sugar water on the tree trunks. Then, very early the next morning, he'd go back and catch the giant beetles eating the sugar water. Today, Dr. Tomo has two dogs, a cat, and a lizard.

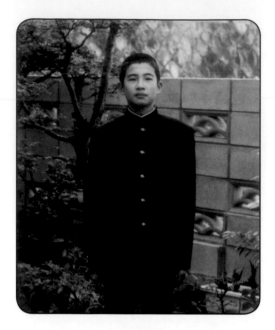

School

School is different in Japan. Starting in the 3rd grade, Dr. Tomo went to public school from 8:00 a.m. to 3:30 p.m. After school, he practiced special writing called calligraphy, took piano lessons, played tennis, and ate dinner. Then, he went back to school to study for an exam to go to a private junior high from 5:00 p.m. to 6:00 p.m. With each grade the evening school lasted longer. In 4th grade, he studied for his exam from 5:00 p.m. to 7:00 p.m., in 5th grade from 5:00 p.m. to 8:00 p.m., and in 6th grade from 5:00 p.m. to 9:00 p.m. He would get home from school at 9:30 p.m. or 10:00 p.m. each night! Dr. Tomo's favorite class in elementary school was music. In junior high, his favorite subject was English. In high school, he didn't like to study anything! He watched a lot of cartoons on TV.

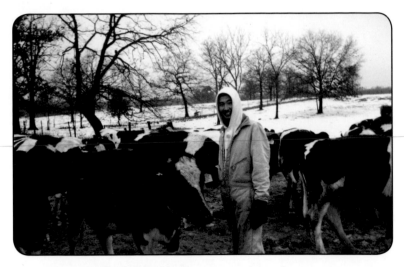

Becoming a veterinarian

Dr. Tomo went to college in the United States at Oklahoma State University. He only spoke Japanese in elementary school so he had to learn English to go to school in the United States. He first wanted to be a flight attendant, but a visit to his roommate's cattle farm changed his mind. He decided to be a veterinarian. Then, there was a problem. Oklahoma State University's veterinary college wouldn't give him an application because he was from Japan. He talked to the dean (principal) of the veterinary school and they decided he could apply. Dr. Tomo was the first student from another country to go to veterinary school in Oklahoma. Dr. Tomo did so well that now the veterinary school welcomes students from all over the world.

Dr. Tomo says:
"Nothing is impossible if you decide to do it."

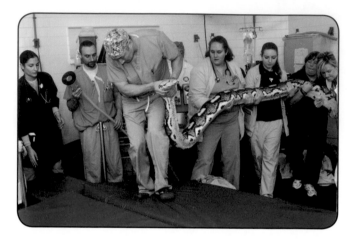

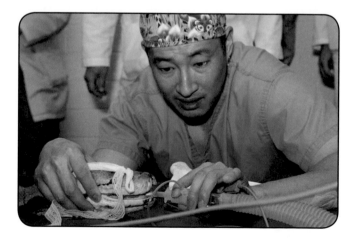

<u>Chapter Two</u>

The Mystery of the Dying Ducks

by Sandy Amass

Dr. Willie Reed woke up at 6:00 a.m. Sammy, his dog, was very excited. She was ready to go outside. Dr. Willie and Sammy went for their morning walk and got the newspaper. Dr. Willie is a husband and father. His son and daughter are all grown up. Dr. Willie lives with his wife, Dr. Dorothy, and his dog, Sammy. After their walk, Dr. Willie, Dr. Dorothy and Sammy all ate breakfast together and caught up on the local news. The news reporter on television said, "Ducks at the local park are dying!" The newspaper reporter wrote, "Isn't it awful that someone is poisoning the ducks at the park!"

Dr. Willie is a veterinarian. He is a diagnostic pathologist. Diagnostic pathologists are like police detectives. When animals die, Dr. Willie must look for clues and solve the mystery of why the animal died. Dr. Willie had a big day ahead of him. He was going to solve the mystery of the dying ducks!

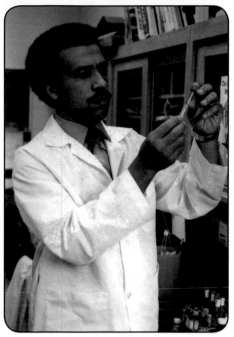

Dr. Willie went to his laboratory. In his laboratory, he examined the dead ducks for clues. He saw that they all had sore throats. "Maybe they are being poisoned," he thought, "or maybe they have a disease." He needed more clues. Next, Dr. Willie took samples from the ducks and looked at them under the microscope. He saw clues that a disease had made the ducks sick. It sure looked like Duck Plague to him! Duck Plague is caused by a virus that can spread quickly and kill many ducks. But, Duck Plague isn't found in the United States. Dr. Willie notified the authorities. He also sent samples to another laboratory to see what they thought. Sure enough, Dr. Willie was right! Duck Plague was in the United States.

Indiana, the state where Dr. Willie lives, has lots and lots of ducks. It was very important to find all of the sick ducks and take care of them right away. Dr. Willie

15

didn't want any more ducks to get sick. He went right to the park to help the ducks. The first step in taking care of the ducks was to catch them. These were wild ducks. They were not pets. Catching them was not going to be easy! Dr. Willie and his team tried to catch the ducks in nets but the ducks just flew onto the lake. The ducks seemed to be laughing at them, "Ha ha, you can't catch us!"

Dr. Willie had a plan. His team would put medicine in the ducks' feed to make the ducks sleepy. Then, his team would collect the sleeping ducks and take care of them. This plan worked well at first. The ducks ate the feed. But then they flew back onto the lake and started to fall asleep! This was an emergency! The ducks had to be saved or they would drown! Dr. Willie looked around and saw a paddleboat. He jumped in the boat with his net and started paddling as fast as he could towards the ducks. Dr. Willie was able to rescue hundreds of ducks that day and take care of them.

Dr. Willie went home happy. It was an exciting day. The next morning Dr. Willie and Sammy went for their walk and got the newspaper. In the newspaper, there was a picture of Dr. Willie wearing his white lab coat, on the paddleboat, saving the ducks.

Meet Dr. Willie Reed

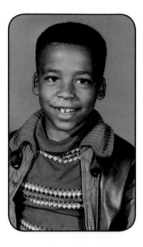

Growing up

Dr. Willie grew up in a small town in southern Alabama called McIntosh. He lived with his father, mother, three younger sisters and his grandmother. His aunts, uncles and another grandmother lived nearby.

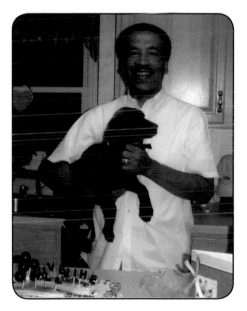

Pets

Dr. Willie grew up around all kinds of animals. His family had horses, cattle, pigs, chickens, turkeys, goats-just about everything. Today, Dr. Willie has Sammy, a chocolate Labrador Retriever, who was given to him as a surprise birthday present.

School

Dr. Willie enjoyed science classes, especially biology, in school. He also loved to read books and short stories in school. Stories by Charles Dickens were his favorite. He would pretend that he was traveling to the places in the books. Every evening after school, Dr. Willie liked to play touch football. In high school, Dr. Willie liked playing the alto saxophone in his high school marching band. He especially liked marching in Mardi Gras parades. Dr. Willie got good grades in high school and graduated at the top of his class. He worked hard in school and it paid off.

Becoming a veterinarian

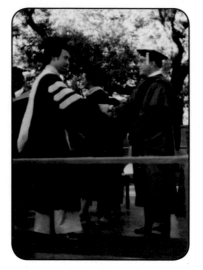

One of Dr. Willie's teachers in high school encouraged him to become a veterinarian. Dr. Willie's father had a strong love for animals and also encouraged a career in veterinary medicine. Dr. Willie went to college and veterinary school at Tuskegee University in Alabama. He always thought that he would come home and be the veterinarian for his hometown. But in veterinary school, Dr. Willie learned about what pathologists do. Dr. Willie decided that he wanted to be a veterinarian who specialized in pathology instead.

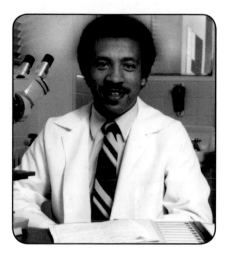

When Dr. Willie went to veterinary school, very few schools in the United States welcomed African Americans. Today, Dr. Willie is Dean of the Purdue University College of Veterinary Medicine. A dean is the principal of the school. Now, Dr. Willie can tell students who want to be veterinarians that they have the opportunity to attend the veterinary school of their choice regardless of the color of their skin.

Dr. Willie says:

"There's nothing wrong with asking for help because there are many great people in the world who are willing to help if you just reach out and ask."

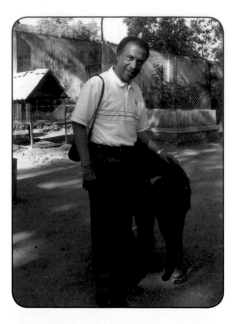

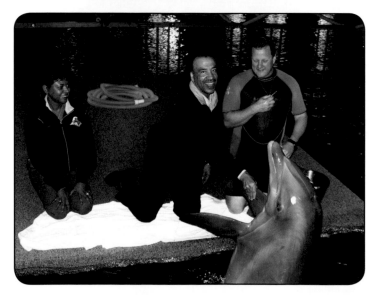

Chapter Three

The Horse Who Stopped Whinnying

by Sandy Amass

Fred is a happy horse. He loves to make a wonderful sound when he is having a really good time. The sound is called a whinny. Fred whinnies all the time. Fred thinks he is a great big horse, but he is a miniature horse. He is the size of a really big dog.

One morning Fred tried to whinny when he saw his family, but a "honk" came out. Then, Fred started having trouble breathing. Something was very wrong. Fred's family took him to the animal hospital.

Dr. Laurent Couëtil is a veterinarian. He is an expert who helps horses who have problems breathing. Dr. Laurent and his wife are early risers. His two sons are in high school. They are just waking up as Dr. Laurent and his wife, Nathalie, grab a cup of coffee and leave to go for their morning swim at the gym. After their workout, they return home for breakfast and watch the morning news. The boys have already eaten and are on their way to school. It is time for Dr. Laurent to start his workday.

Dr. Laurent arrives at the animal hospital. He meets with the students and the other veterinarians. They talk about each animal that is in the hospital. They talk about how the animal is feeling and what treatments it might need. They talk about which animals are all better and can go home. Then, they meet with the families that have brought new animals in for an appointment. Dr. Laurent's first patient of the day is Fred.

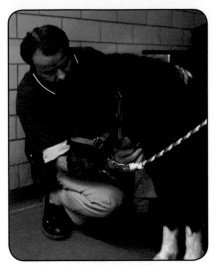

Dr. Laurent met Fred's family and examined Fred. Fred's honk was coming from his throat. The honk got louder when Fred got excited and quieter when Fred calmed down. Dr. Laurent needed to see what was happening in Fred's throat so he took Fred down the hall to see veterinarians who specialize in taking radiographs (x rays).

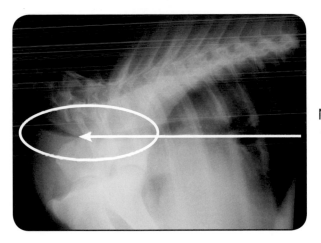

Narrowing windpipe

The radiographs showed that Fred had a collapsed windpipe. The windpipe (or trachea) is the tube that brings air to the lungs. Sometimes animals are born with a windpipe that has a problem. When the animal gets older, the problem causes the windpipe to collapse and the animal will have trouble breathing. In regular-sized horses, there is a surgery to fix the windpipe. But that surgery would not work for Fred, since Fred was so small. Then, Dr. Laurent read about a new procedure that helped people who had collapsed windpipes. He called his friend who was a physician (people doctor) to see if the procedure for people might help Fred. They decided it would.

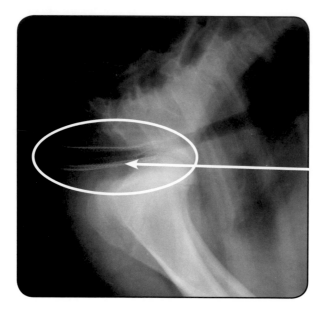

Tube in Fred's windpipe

The new procedure involved putting a tube inside Fred's windpipe so it would not collapse. A team of experts was called in because this was the first time the procedure would be done on a horse. Veterinary anesthesiologists, like Dr. Tomo, came in to make sure

Fred was asleep during surgery and did not feel any pain. Veterinarians who specialized in taking radiographs were called in to make sure they put the tube in the right place. Veterinary technicians came in to make sure everything went smoothly. Finally, Dr. Laurent and his friend the physician were there to perform the procedure. They used a tool called an endoscope to put the tube in Fred's windpipe. An endoscope is long instrument that can be moved around like a snake. Using an endoscope is like playing a video game. Dr. Laurent used a controller to pick up the tube with the endoscope, slide the tube down Fred's nose and into his windpipe, and then place the tube in the right spot in Fred's windpipe.

After the procedure, Fred was moved to a special room where he could wake up safely. Soon, Fred opened his eyes and looked at the medical team surrounding him. Then, Fred started whinnying! Everyone cheered! He was a happy horse again!

Dr. Laurent finished up his day working with students and the veterinary team to make sure the animal patients staying overnight had everything they needed. Then, he went home and told his family about the great day that he had.

Meet Dr. Laurent Couëtil

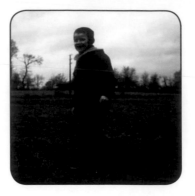

Growing up

Dr. Laurent grew up in the Normandy region of France with his parents and younger sister. They had a farm with a few cattle and many horses. Dr. Laurent's father passed away when Dr. Laurent was 7 years old. Dr. Laurent spent most of his time helping his mom at the farm.

Pets

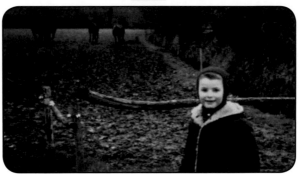

Dr. Laurent grew up around the horses and cattle on his family's farm. He also had two dogs and a cat that lived outside. Dr. Laurent loved riding horses. He would ride race horses and show horses. He loved jumping!

School

Dr. Laurent loved science classes and reading in school. He also enjoyed learning Spanish. Dr. Laurent did well in school. He was always one of the top three students in his high school class. After school, Dr. Laurent liked to play soccer, ride bikes, and read comic books. Dr. Laurent grew up close to the ocean. He learned to wind surf when he was a teenager and enjoyed windsurfing and sailing.

Becoming a veterinarian

When Dr. Laurent was growing up, he got along well with the veterinarian that would come and take care of his family's horses. The veterinarian would take him along when he visited other farms. When Dr. Laurent was 14 or 15 years old, he decided to be a veterinarian. His biggest challenge was that his family was poor and veterinary school was expensive. He was able to get financial help so that he could afford to go to school. He went to veterinary school in Paris, France.

Dr. Laurent was a veterinarian in France for a while. Then, he decided that he wanted to specialize in taking care of horses. He moved to the United States and went to Tufts University to become an equine (horse) sports medicine specialist. Now, Dr. Laurent is a teacher at the Purdue University College of Veterinary Medicine. He loves to help horses and teach students how they can best take care of their animal patients.

Dr. Laurent says:
"Be true to yourself and honest."

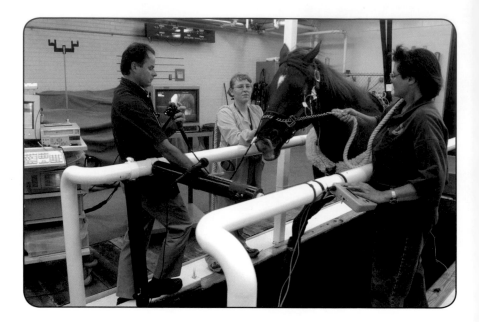

<u>Chapter Four</u>

The Vemulapalli Veterinarians

by Paula Green and Kauline Davis

Animals Helping People

Dr. Tracy Vemulapalli (Vem-ooh-lah-pah-lee) is in charge of all the animals that live at the veterinary school. Researchers work with these animals to learn more about helping animals and people live better, healthier lives.

The technicians, Dr. Tracy's helpers, help her find out whether or not an animal is sick and needs medication. She also helps teach veterinary students about bacteriology (germs) and whether or not an animal is healthy and can contribute to research. She has a lot of other responsibilities at the veterinary school.

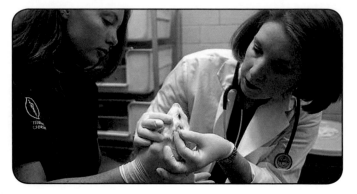

When a veterinarian wants to do research they are usually trying to find out ways to cure a disease. An important part of Dr. Tracy's job is to make sure the animals they are working with are healthy before they begin any research and to provide veterinary care for the animals during the research.

Much of the research that Dr. Tracy helps other doctors do is trying to find treatments for human diseases, such as diabetes. You may know a person or an animal that has diabetes. Much of the research in veterinary medicine is done to help improve the lives of people by curing and properly treating different diseases first in animals.

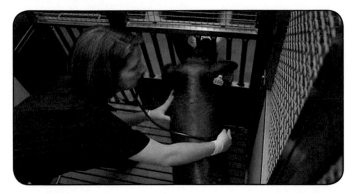

Dr. Tracy's day starts off the same way every day. She has two children, a 12 year old and a 5 year old, and so the morning is spent making sure everyone has properly dressed, eaten breakfast, packed their bookbags, and gotten off to school. Some mornings are pretty hectic.

Once at work, Dr. Tracy meets with her technicians and they make sure the animals are taken care of and are well so that the researchers can begin their day.

At the end of a work day, Dr. Tracy checks that all the animals in the hospital have been properly taken care of. She prepares for the next day's lesson for her students and then she heads for home. She picks up her kids from school, checks their homework, prepares dinner, takes them to their different practices, takes care of the family pets, and gets ready for the next day.

However, one evening just as everyone was ready to leave, a big dog came in with a bite in his abdomen (belly) from a much smaller dog that it lived with. It seemed that the two dogs had a fight and the smaller dog had enough so he bit his friend! At first, the bite wound did not look very deep, so Dr. Tracy sent all of her assistants home. To her surprise, when she returned to the examination room and looked closer at the bite, she realized the dog's wound was so deep that his insides were trying to come outside!

After putting his organs back into place inside his belly all by herself, she sutured (sewed up) his wound, gave him pain medication, and hoped for the best. That was the most surprising and coolest case Dr. Tracy had ever had. It is also her biggest success story. That dog lived a long time after that adventure. Dr. Tracy did a great job!

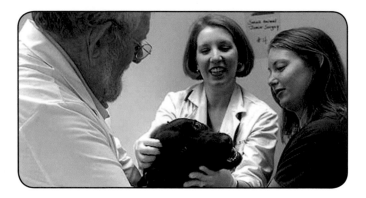

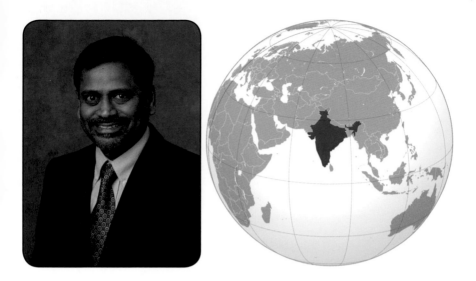

The Famous Chicken Vet (Who Married Dr. Tracy)

Dr. Ramesh Vemulapalli was concerned. He was a new graduate of veterinary school and the newest veterinarian in his practice, when he was faced with a big problem of dying birds on a chicken farm in India. The farmer had a pretty large farm of about 5,000 chickens, and the birds had started dying the day before at an alarming rate of 10 birds per hour. By the time Dr. Ramesh talked to the farmer that morning, at least 100 birds had died! The farmer was very concerned about this. There were two senior veterinarians in the practice, but they were not available to go to the farm. The farmer sent a car to pick up Dr. Ramesh to see if he could figure out what was going on and prevent any more birds from dying. When Dr. Ramesh arrived at the farm he knew he didn't have a lot of time to figure out the problem by doing lots of tests. To make things worse, it was the holiday season in India so many places would be closed. Dr.

Ramesh performed necropsies (examined dead birds) and saw signs of an infection. The sick birds that were still alive had fevers. He thought to himself, "This must be a blood infection of some sort, but what is causing it?" With no time to run tests, Dr. Ramesh called up the local drug store and asked them what medicine was in stock and available now. The store had a new medicine available. Dr. Ramesh purchased a whole bunch of it and had several farm workers help him begin treating the birds with this powerful antibiotic (drug used to kill germs) immediately. Within the next eight hours, the birds started doing much better, and there were no more deaths. Dr. Ramesh became quite popular after that. Even though he was the "kid" at the practice where he worked, all the farmers around who heard the story of how he saved this flock would ask for him by name whenever they needed a veterinarian!

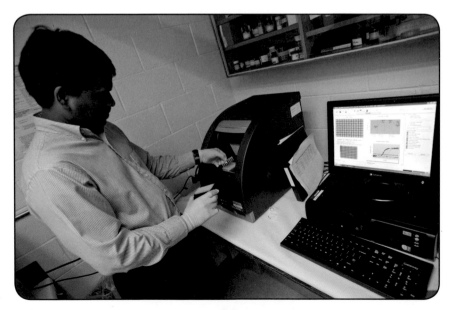

Dr. Ramesh had a lot of fun practicing poultry (chicken) medicine in India. He enjoyed traveling from farm to farm on his motorcycle. He helped farmers come up with new and better ways to keep their chickens healthy and lay more eggs. Sometimes Dr. Ramesh had to treat many birds on many farms when there was an outbreak of an infection; those times were not so much fun. Cell phones were not popular back then, so instead of calling the farmers, Dr. Ramesh had to travel to each farm to warn the owners of the outbreak in the area. He would bring antibiotics that could be given to the chickens in their water or feed, or given as a shot to individual birds.

Even though he really liked practicing poultry medicine in India, eventually Dr. Ramesh began to miss… something. At first he tried learning about raising chickens, but he only did that for a year, deciding he wasn't really cut out for that. Then he realized he missed studying, and having new and different problems to solve. So he decided to return to school, get a Masters degree in Animal Biochemistry, and work in a university or college. He did return to school and got his Master's degree, but he was unable to get a job in India when he graduated.

His father and friends encouraged him to go to school in the United States and get his Ph.D. His school counselor in India also encouraged him, saying he had great abilities when it came to research. His family had no money to support this, so Dr. Ramesh looked for research jobs to get money for his education. He got good grades on the tests he needed for attending graduate school in the United States. He was accepted into a Ph.D. program at University of Maryland, College Park to do research on equine (horse) diseases. He was excited about this because he really liked working with horses.

At the University of Maryland, College Park, Dr. Ramesh worked on a disease of horses called Potomac Horse Fever. This disease was a huge problem for horses particularly in the Washington, D.C. area where the Potomac River is present, and that's where the disease gets its name. Potomac Horse Fever is caused by a germ called *Neorickettsia risticii*. Horses with this disease get fever and diarrhea. Sometimes there are other problems, such as colic (stomach ache), arthritis (joint pain and swelling), and lameness (limping). Antibiotics were used to treat this disease, but were only effective if the disease was caught early enough, so a quick test for *Neorickettsia risticii* was needed in order to treat these horses early enough to help them get better.

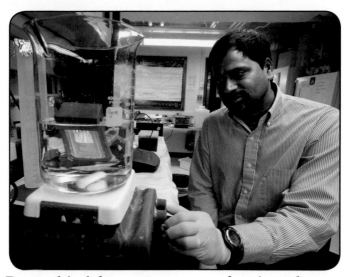

Dr. Ramesh's laboratory team developed a test and offered that test to the equine veterinarians in the area. They used the results of the test for their research. At the time, Dr. Ramesh and his team were the only ones providing this test, and they did it for free because they used the results to help learn more about the germ and how to stop it from making horses sick. The equine veterinarians took blood samples from sick horses, and Dr. Ramesh brought them back to the lab to run the test on them. The results of the test were ready in the middle of the night and Dr. Ramesh gave the results to the equine veterinarians early the next morning. Dr. Ramesh got a lot of satisfaction by being so helpful to the equine veterinarians and the sick horses. Best of all, the equine veterinarians would often treat Dr. Ramesh to lunch!

After the first year in his Ph.D. program, Dr. Ramesh had to work as a teaching assistant to get enough money to pay for school. At first he was really upset about this, thinking about all the time he would have to spend teaching when he could be doing research. However, he soon found out that he really enjoyed teaching, and that teaching helped him to speak English better; he learned the correct pronunciation of many words. Dr. Ramesh continued to be a teaching assistant for the next 4 years while finishing his Ph.D. research, and that gave him the practice and confidence to become a really great teacher. The best part about his teaching job at the University of Maryland was that he met his wife, Dr. Tracy, while working there.

Meet Dr. Tracy and Dr. Ramesh

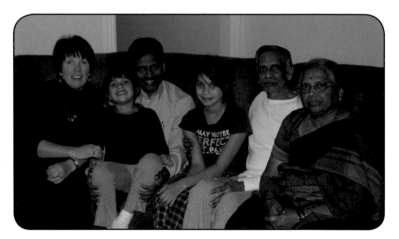

Growing up

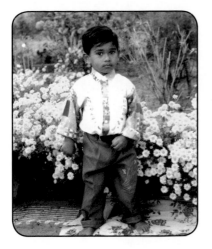 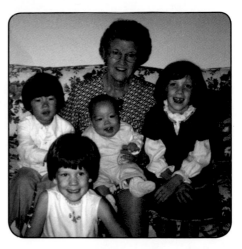

Dr. Tracy grew up in Elkton, Maryland in a very "international" family. The eldest of four children, she has a younger sister and two younger brothers. Her brothers are from South Korea. Dr. Ramesh grew up on his parents' farm outside the village of Kancharlapalem in the state of Andra Pradesh in India. He liked to explore the wilderness surrounding the farm.

Dr. Ramesh was the youngest of three children. He has an older brother and an older sister. Because cameras were very expensive when he was a boy, Dr. Ramesh doesn't have any pictures of himself when he was a kid. However, he looked just like his nephew (pictured on left).

Today, Drs. Ramesh and Tracy are two busy veterinarians who both work at Purdue University and are the proud parents of two wonderful daughters.

Pets

Growing up, Dr. Ramesh always had dogs as pets. Also, every calf that was born on the farm was a pet until it got too big.

Dr. Tracy had a cat, several goldfish, and a ferret when she was a kid. Some people thought Dr. Tracy's ferret was a bit stinky, but she thought her ferret smelled "just fine"! Today, Drs. Ramesh and Tracy have a dog, two cats, four goldfish, and a betta fish.

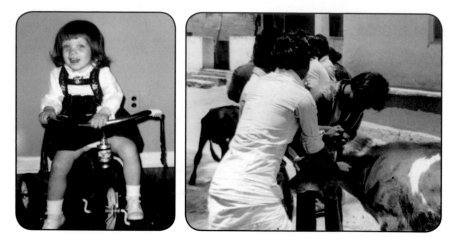

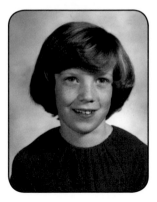 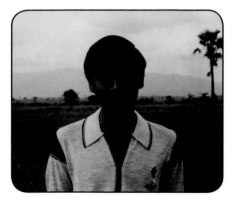

School

Dr. Tracy's favorite subjects in school were science, math, history, and art. Dr. Tracy loved to read. Her favorite books to read were mysteries. They inspired her to be a veterinarian. She liked the idea of solving mysteries to find out why an animal was sick and how to make it better.

Dr. Ramesh's favorite subjects in school were math, physics, and chemistry. He was a Boy Scout in middle and high school. One of his favorite summertime activities was climbing up mango trees and eating the mangos.

Becoming a veterinarian

Dr. Ramesh decided to go to veterinary school after high school because he didn't want to be a physician. In India, you go to veterinary school right after high school. Dr. Ramesh went to the College of Veterinary Sciences in Tirupati in Andra Pradesh, India. Today, Dr. Ramesh is in charge of an entire department at Purdue University's College of Veterinary Medicine. He is an expert on making better tests to detect diseases and better vaccines (shots) to prevent diseases.

Dr. Tracy was in the 5th grade when she decided to become a veterinarian. She found some courses in college were easy and some were hard. When she had a course that was hard, she would ask her teachers and classmates for help. Dr. Tracy went to veterinary school at Virginia-Maryland Regional College of Veterinary Medicine (Virginia Tech).

Dr. Tracy says

"Ask for help and work hard and you'll see good results."

Dr. Ramesh says

"Be passionate about what you do, and never EVER give up!"

Chapter Five

A Broken Heart
by Kauline Davis

Pixie is a Papillon. Papillons are a breed of small dogs. Pixie was sad. She couldn't run and play with the other dogs because she was born with a heart problem. Pixie's problem is called Patent Ductus Arteriosus. Lots of animal species can have this problem, and it can also be seen in children. Patent Ductus Arteriosus happens when a blood vessel (duct) in the heart that is supposed to close off after an animal is born, doesn't close.

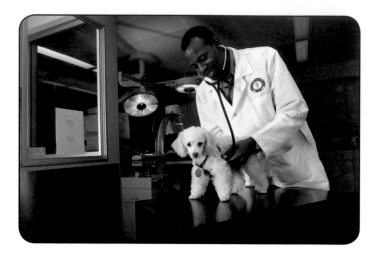

This morning, Pixie is going to see Dr. Henry Green. Dr. Henry is a veterinary cardiologist. That means he specializes in diseases of the heart. He is the first African-American veterinarian in the United States to be board-certified in cardiology. Veterinarians who become board certified study extra hard and have to take a special test. If they pass, they are experts in their area. There are only about 200 veterinarians who are heart specialists in the entire country! Dr. Henry loves all the different aspects of his job. He loves teaching students, he loves working on research that will help animals as well as humans, and he loves seeing his animal patients in the clinic.

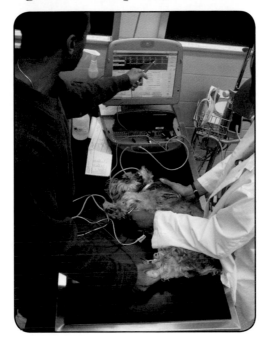

On days when Dr. Henry is scheduled to be in the clinic, he works with students who want to be veterinarians and veterinary nurses. He also works with residents (veterinarians who want to be specialists). The students and residents meet the pet owners and perform examinations on the pets, then Dr. Henry goes over the cases with them. This is a very important part of teaching future veterinarians. Students are able to see clients, order the right tests, and develop a treatment plan, all under the supervision of an experienced veterinarian like Dr. Henry. Some of the tests Dr. Henry and his team might use to learn about the hearts of his patients include taking radiographs and performing ultrasounds of the heart.

Another important part of Dr. Henry's job is his research. When he isn't working in the clinic, he focuses on his research projects by writing up results and designing and performing new experiments and procedures. Dr. Henry is part of a team of researchers who work mostly with pacemakers and develop other ways to solve heart disease problems in dogs. Pacemakers help the dog's heart beat properly. When Dr. Henry and his team began having so much success helping small dogs, they asked the question "maybe this can work in babies?" So they teamed up with pediatricians and began working to see if some of the procedures they had used in dogs would be safe for human babies suffering from the same heart conditions.

Today, Dr. Henry and his team fixed Pixie's heart using a surgery that Dr. Henry helped develop. The surgery closed off the duct so Pixie's heart will work again. Dr. Henry and his colleagues were particularly excited about Pixie since she was the smallest dog on which they had ever performed this surgery!

After surgery, Dr. Henry and his team happily sent Pixie home with her family. It was a great day!

Meet Dr. Henry Green

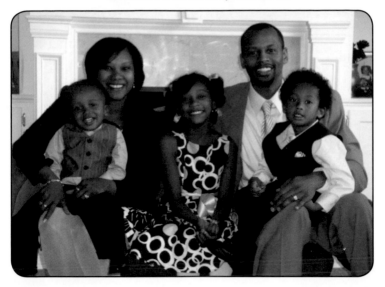

Growing Up

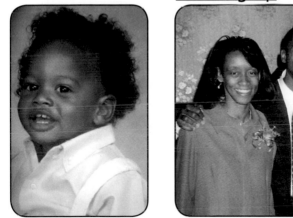

Dr. Henry grew up in the 9th ward of New Orleans, Louisiana. He was fortunate to have a village of people to help raise him, and his mentors were his mom and dad. Today, Dr. Henry is married and a father of three small children. Dr. Henry's wife, Mrs. Paula Green, is

47

also a busy professional and works as a high-school counselor. Every day, Dr. Henry begins his day early by getting the Green kids ready for school and day care, and he drops them off before heading to the clinic. There are many days that Dr. Henry might have to work late at the clinic, monitoring his patients, but he always takes a break during the early evening to go home and play with his children, coach his daughter's basketball team, take one of his sons to T-ball practice, or even cook dinner. Dr. Henry is a great cook!

Pets

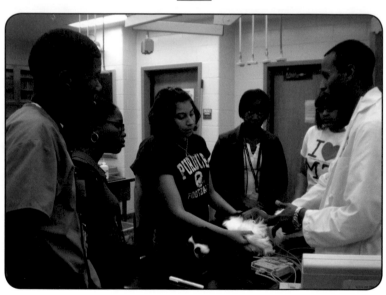

Today, Dr. Henry's family has a pet dog, a Cavalier King Charles Spaniel, named "Ozzie."

School

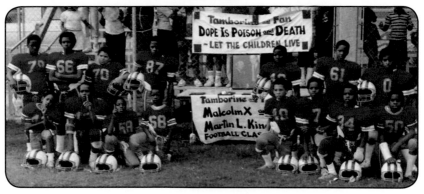

When Dr. Henry was a kid, he loved reading science and history books. He often wrote plays, which his mother would edit and keep in a special book. Dr. Henry also LOVED playing sports. Almost every day, he played or practiced some sport such as football, baseball, or track. Even when it was raining outside, Dr. Henry and his sisters would find a way to make a sport-like competition inside. For example, they bent wire clothes hangers to make basketball goals out of them. Then they would tear old shirts and tie strips to the hanger to give the appearance of the nets and hang the goals in the doorway. They would use a pair of rolled up socks as the ball and have an indoor "basketball" game. They also liked to play sports video games on the computer.

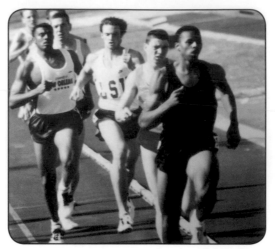

Dr. Henry always tells his students that one of the most important things you can do is to take your education seriously. He believes it is truly valuable to know how to do things, and to understand why things happen.

<u>Becoming a veterinarian</u>

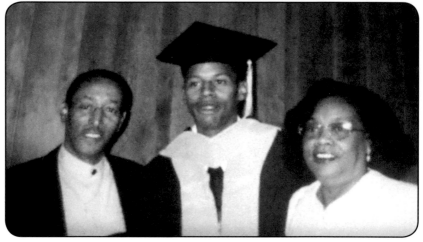

Growing up in the inner city, Dr. Henry did not have the same exposure to veterinary medicine that say kids on a farm might have, but his grandmother raised

German Shepherd Dogs and he was always impressed by the veterinarian who took care of those dogs. He wanted to be a veterinarian since the 6th grade. Dr. Henry went to college at the University of New Orleans. Then, he attended Louisiana State University College of Veterinary Medicine.

Dr. Henry comes from a family of educators, so it's no surprise that he loves to teach! Dr. Henry teaches cardiology classes to veterinary students before they enter their 4th year, which is when they get to work in the clinic and see patients. One of the things he loves about teaching is the fact that he gets to find new and interesting ways to explain concepts that many students may find difficult to understand. When a student finally "gets it", or understands a key point that Dr. Henry has been trying to explain, he feels a huge sense of accomplishment, and satisfaction. Dr. Henry feels happy when a student learns something important that he or she was struggling to understand.

Dr. Henry says:

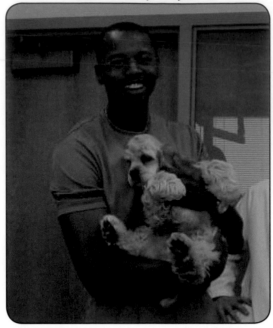

"A thirst for learning is the best thing you can have," says Dr. Henry. "There is always something new to discover, and without the desire to learn we would settle for a lot of things, and we wouldn't question if we could make things better." Dr. Henry believes we can always make things better!

<u>Chapter Six</u>

Crime Scene Investigator

by Paula Green

Dr. Yava Jones is a veterinary pathologist. She teaches, does research and performs diagnostic services. She does necropsies which means she does examinations on animals that have died.

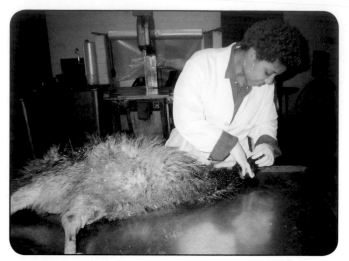

Most days Dr. Yava has to drag herself out of bed because after a long day at work, she usually exercises and then stays up late reading or watching TV.

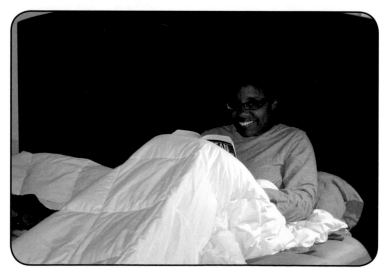

Once at work Dr. Yava gets a hot cup of coffee, goes to her office, reviews mail and email, reviews cases, plans lessons, and gets ready for the rest of her day.

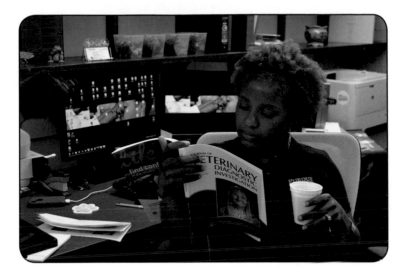

Some mornings Dr. Yava teaches a class to veterinary students. She teaches the students how to determine what type of diseases an animal may have had or what actually caused the animal to die.

In the afternoon (1:00 p.m.), Dr. Yava begins the necropsy service. She reviews cases with veterinary students by examining the tissue and organs of the deceased animal.

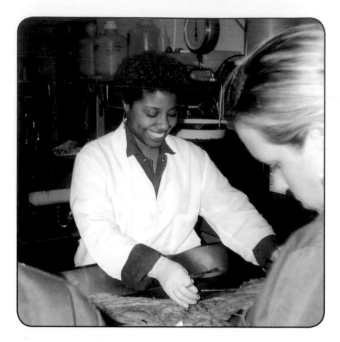

The necropsy examination rooms are extremely cold to prevent the germs from all of the dead animals from growing. So everyone is also very cold while doing the necropsies. It is worse in winter, as you can imagine.

The team does all the cases for that day, opening up all the animals (chest, stomach) with a large knife, to see if any of their organs have disease. They take samples of each organ and send those samples to all of the laboratories so they can test for bacteria, viruses or see if the animal digested any kind of toxic (poisonous) substance. They also put tissues in formalin to preserve them so they can look at them under the microscope. Examining the tissue under the microscope allows pathologists to confirm the diagnosis they suspected on the necropsy.

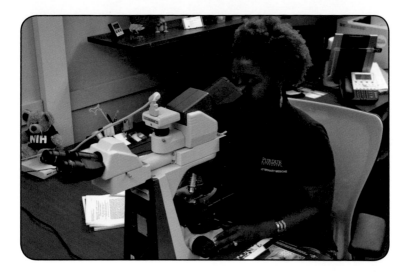

Why do pathologists do this? It helps the owner of the animal understand what caused the death of their animal. One case like this was the death of a horse. The neighbor of the horse's owner, thought she was starving the horse because it looked under nourished (extremely thin and unhealthy looking). The neighbor reported the owner to the authorities when the horse died.

To prove that she didn't mistreat her horse, the owner submitted the horse for necropsy to find out what happened to her dear animal. Upon the initial examination, the horse's stomach was empty and had a really low fat percentage which suggested starvation. Was the owner feeding the horse or not? After further examination, Dr. Yava discovered the liver tissue had a tumor. Liver cancer was the reason the animal was not eating and was the true culprit. The owner was found innocent! You can say Dr. Yava runs the Crime Scene Investigation (CSI) Unit of veterinary medicine.

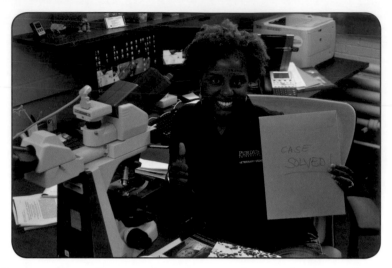

Some days the work may not be as intense but the location may be. As an Army veterinary reservist, Dr. Yava took care of the military dogs that were deployed with the Army to Afghanistan.

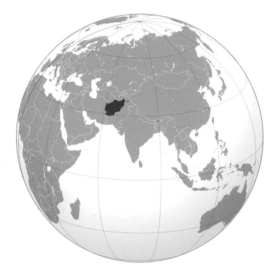

Dr. Yava also worked with the medical corps during their humanitarian mission to local villages. While the medics took care of the people, Dr. Yava gave shots to animals that needed them and performed examinations on the local pets. She was even asked to examine a chicken by one little girl.

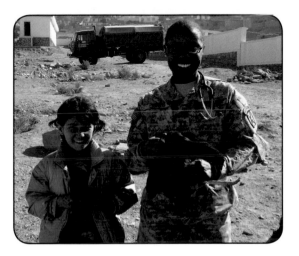

The day can bring all kinds of cases and surprises. Dr. Yava is happy that her job allows her to bring smiles and peace of mind to the people she serves.

Dr. Yava's cases are quiet so she usually needs to do something that is a bit more lively and active-get it? At the end of the day, she goes to the gym and works out.

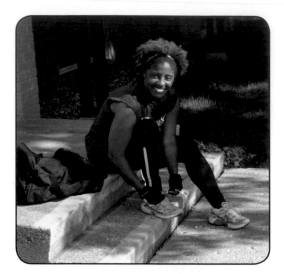

Once at home, she prepares a meal and watches TV.

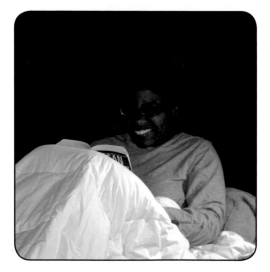

Meet Dr. Yava Jones

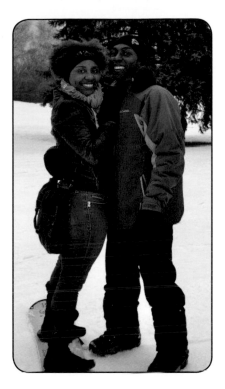

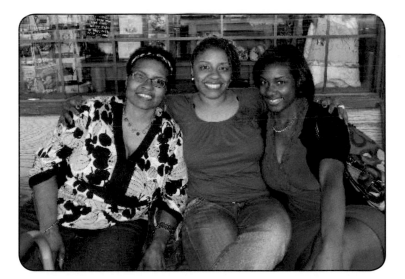

Growing Up

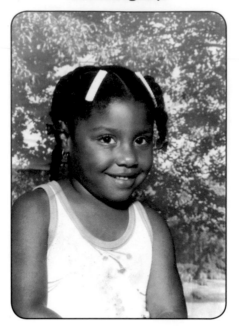

Dr. Yava grew up in a mostly rural area in Childersburg, Alabama. For most of her childhood, her mother raised her as a single parent. Her mother and father divorced when Dr. Yava was a toddler, but she is still close to her dad. Dr. Yava has a little sister who is 11 years younger than her. So Dr. Yava was both a big sister and surrogate mother for her little sister because their mom worked a lot. They also spent a lot of time at their grandmother's house since she lived nearby. The military has always been an important part of Dr. Yava's life. Her mom was in the Air Force, her dad was in the Army, and her grandpa was also in the Air Force. Dr. Yava is engaged to be married to her fiancé, Mr. Jason who also works at Purdue as an engineer.

Pets

Dr. Yava had a German Shepherd Dog named Bandit growing up. Today she has a cat named Sophie, and three fish, Ivy, Goldie, and Blackie.

School

Dr. Yava's favorite subject in school was Science. She liked to read and hang with her friends. She read a lot. Dr. Yava loved mystery books! In high school, she played sports. Softball and volleyball were her favorites but she also played basketball. She also played volleyball in college.

Becoming a veterinarian

Dr. Yava went to college a year early. She joined the Army Reserves while she was in college. She was also in the Upward Bound Program. Mentors in the program showed her what an African American professional could look like and achieve. She always wanted to be a veterinarian, but she didn't really know any veterinarians or have any veterinarian role models. Mentors in the Upward Bound Program introduced her to the first African American veterinarian she'd ever met. Her biggest challenge was lack of experience when applying to vet school. But, she did have other things: leadership, lots of activities in her community, and good grades! Dr. Yava went to veterinary school at Tuskegee University. She went on to complete a residency in veterinary pathology and a Ph.D. in pathology at Michigan State University. Today, she is a board-certified veterinary pathologist.

Dr. Yava says:

"Don't let where you came from dictate where you will go."

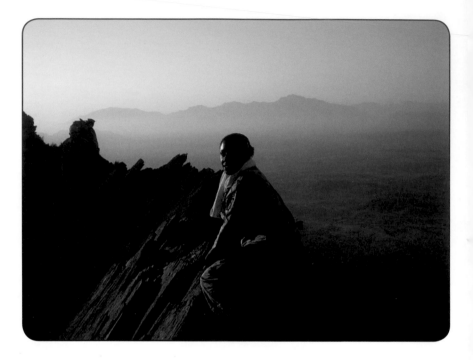

This is a picture of Dr. Yava on top of the Ghar Mountain in Kabul, Afghanistan.